Love 'N' Birth

When Birth Calls:

Developing Your Inner Birthworker

"Dedicated to Black Women who are seeking guidance on their path to becoming a Birthworker"

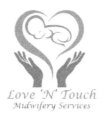

Love 'N' Touch
Midwifery Services

Written by Sekesa Berry

Cover Art by Y'Na Snipes Evans

i

Love 'N' Birth, When Birth Calls.: Developing Your Inner Birthworker
Revised Edition
Written by Sekesa Berry
Edited by Amunet Berry-Blunt
Cover Art by Y'Na Snipes Evans, Art of Business dba YNaDesigns
Cover Image, "African American Midwife Maude Callen Delivering a Baby" by W.
Eugene Smith, 1951 "

Email: info@loventouch.com
Website: www.loventouch.com

Love 'N' Birth

When Birth Calls:

Developing Your Inner Birthworker

Contents

Foreword

Introduction

Becoming a Birthworker

What is a Doula?

Types of Labor Assistants (Doulas)

What is a Birth Assistant?

What is an Obstetrician?

What is a Midwife?

Pathways to Midwifery

Closing Remind-hers

About the Author

Foreword

Sekesa Berry has been my sister and friend for over twelve years. Our bond was instantly established on the foundation of Black Womanhood, Indigenous Spirituality, Supportive Sisterhood, Natural Birthing, Motherhood and the Wholistic rearing of our children, and continued personal growth and evolution. These are also the core principles she implements in the work that she does as a doula and midwife. This, I know for sure. And this is what made it clear that she was the sure fit to usher my 5th child into the world...even though she herself wasn't quite sure at that time.

That home birth experience elevated my dear friend from doula to midwife. I had every confidence in Sekesa's competence, skill set, vibratory essence, and problem-solving abilities to make my birth experience what I wanted and needed it to be. As a mother of six naturally birthed children (3 of which were home births), I can confidently say that Sekesa is my go-to person when I or my friends need information and suggestions on issues of conception, gestation, post-partum, newborn babies, lactation, child development and so much more! She has caught many of the babies in my community and the Mamas all share the same sentiment. To date, she has facilitated two of my births, and if I ever have another child, Sekesa is the one midwife I will call upon. She has and continues to put in the work, the study, the sweat, time and sometimes tears. And now her words...these words that you will read in this book, will surely enlighten, and enrich your journey. May you be blessed and inspired by this work!

Tamara Nichita Simmons-Bush,
Each One Teach One Educational Services
November 19, 2018

Introduction

My inspiration for writing this book comes from my personal challenges while developing my inner Birthworker. During my process I always knew my destination was Midwifery, yet I struggled to decide exactly how I would travel towards the title. My spirit wrestled with reasoning, for treading the paved path lined with flowers (and hidden thorns) or voyage the trail overgrown with weeds. One path appearing attractive but required caution; the other path looked neglected and required great maintenance. My heart guided my steps with passion while my ancestors held my hands and pulled me along the path less traveled, with promise of purpose and strides of legacy along the way.

Within my years of determination to answer an inner calling and gifted birth right to serving women, I have received battle scars of disapproval by some and war injuries of distrust by others. There have been casualties of divorces and heartbreaks of lovers lost. I have experienced many isolating challenges and frightening circumstances. Yet I prevailed in my journey! To this truth I stand, rooted in the traditions and indigenous practices of Traditional Midwifery. Only to reach my destination with the knowing that my being, in the sheroic powers that have possessed, serves as a threat to modern medicine and an embarrassment to the evolving Midwifery status quo.

I wrote this book to provide guidance based on my personal and professional experience of blazing an overgrown trail into Traditional Midwifery. It has been both a frustrating and exhilarating, long walk to the title of Midwife. Which in turn grants me great honor and pride. In Birthwork I can honestly say that I have seen many called, yet so few are chosen.

I wrote this for my sistars who hear the call to Birthwork and seeking guidance and answers. Within these pages you will prayerfully find arrows, road signs and streetlights to make your journey towards developing your Inner Birthworker more clear and direct.

What is a Birthworker?

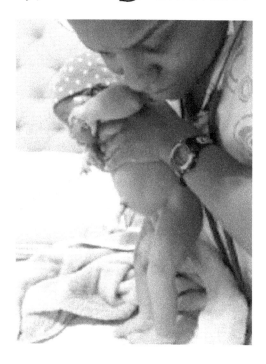

Birthworker is a relatively new term to describe one who works within the maternal field during the childbearing period. It can include Obstetricians, Midwives, Labor & Delivery Nurses, Birth Assistants and Doulas. The term is often inclusive of Childbirth Educators, Placenta Encapsulators, Breastfeeding Counselors and Lactation Consultants as well. I recall the first time I used this term in 2010 while teaching a breastfeeding class to aspiring doulas. I introduced myself as a Birthworker because at the time I was disassociating with the word doula. I also needed my title to include that I was a Breastfeeding Counselor as well. So, it felt suitable to refer to myself as a Birthworker. I don't recall hearing the term prior to that day. I also recall explaining it to people every time I said it. I would always say that because I service both breast and bottom it is easier to call myself a Birthworker. Now, much like the word doula, it is evolving into a very common term.

For the duration of this book, the word Doula is interchanged with Labor Assistant, which is fitting since labor literally means physically hard work. Defining Labor Assistant as one who assists with work.

A Labor of Love

The idea of doing birthwork can be highly praised by some and disgusting to others. I have often said that birthwork is a glorified title and dirty work. Ultimately, I'm certain that any Birthworker will agree that this profession is a labor of love. It can be long hours, sleepless nights, foul smells, gory scenes and, in some cases, unhappy endings. So why would any sane person want to subject themselves to this kind of work? For me, birth is intoxicating! I am honestly addicted! I love knowing that I played a small role in an epic event such as the birth of a new baby and welcoming another ancestor.

Conception and birth is often taken for granted in today's busy society. However, when we consider the natural biological barriers designed to prevent the sperm from ever meeting the egg, and the countless possibilities for genetic mutation, then every conception is truly immaculate, and every birth of a healthy baby is a miracle.

Aside from the gory scenes and foul smells, birthwork is exciting, spontaneous, beautiful, and fulfilling. Birthwork demands flexibility and adaptability. You must be able to immediately assess an unplanned situation and respond responsibly. A mother may sit on the toilet to relieve herself and out comes a baby. You may be expecting a head and out comes a foot! My favorite is when you check a mom (cervical exam) and she is 4-5cm and two surges later she is completely dilated (10cm) and baby is born. Even within hospitals, where there is great effort to micromanage birth, uneventful dynamics can and do occur. I have unexpectedly caught a couple of babies serving as the Labor Assistant in a hospital.

Birthwork is completely life-altering. It can make scheduling events challenging. An on-call window for an independent, homebirth Midwife is about five weeks, from 37 until 42+ weeks. For a Labor Assistant it is any day from the time of being hired, because if the mother enters labor pre-term, then the Labor Assistant is expected to be present. We, as independent contractors, can be present at a birth for two plus days, so as Birthworkers we quickly learn to carry extra clothes and our birthing supplies in the car. My children have grown into our lifestyle, and even my extended family members. It's comical to hear them prelude event-planning with me by first saying, "If you're not on-call for a birth......" This lifestyle can also impact your availability and your presence at special events such as weddings, birthday celebrations, award ceremonies, etcetera, so planning ahead is super important!

This same absence and inconvenient lifestyle can be taxing on marriage and intimate relationships. Even those that service in the hospital can be on-call 2-4-day rotations when they are strictly at the hospital for anyone that is admitted for birth. If your marriage or significant relationship is already fragile - meaning, you're having problems - then now is not the time to enter birthwork! It is better to resolve those disputes and establish a solid bond. You will need your partner to be supportive and encouraging in this endeavor. You also need to be intentional about scheduling special time just for them. Having a functional and cooperative support system as well as reliable backup is critical to your success as a Birthworker. Specifically, if you are doing this work as a primary source of income.

Work Smart!!

Paradigm of Birth

The polar opposite of control (manage, govern, regulate) is release (relief, freedom, relax). One action cannot exist in the presence of the other. In order to release, you are no longer in control, and vice versa. Yet there is an irony in this concept that is revealed in both meditation and birth. Mediation is the art of releasing and letting go, however it requires more muscles in the hueman body than any other exercise. Meditation requires complete self-control inwardly while releasing control outwardly (control of your surroundings). Birth is a type of meditation! It requires a complete release of self-control inwardly as not to hold tension and minimize resistance within the body, while maintaining control over your physical reactions outwardly.

Birthwork has a similar paradigm. Self-control within a birthing space is critical. You must refrain from projecting your thoughts, feelings, and desires on the family that you are serving. All while remaining calm, supportive, and most importantly, non-judgmental.

January 5th, 2010: A Test of Self-Control

I met her in a space of high inner-G and strong confidence. She was a vegetarian and prided herself on eating clean and healthy. She kept an immaculate home, surrounded by African art and meditative tools. She claimed this birth as, "birthing her inner child". Her first birth was via cesarean, and she felt compelled to birth this baby naturally. I was sure this would be a smooth VBAC homebirth experience.

I arrived early in her labor, a day prior to birth. It presented with scattered and inconsistent surges that appeared to be intense. We walked, talked, had breakfast and lunch together alongside her Midwife. We danced and watched TV while working through her surges as they would increase then decrease. As the moon grew high, the mommy's surges grew more intense and regular. Throughout the night I watched her mentally slow down her labor and allow fear to creep into her thoughts.

It was unbelievable and unacceptable to me! I thought that I could convince her of her power by speaking positive affirmations to her, such as: you can do this mommy, your powerful, your strong, your body was meant to birth this baby. I consistently attempted to remind her of her previous reasoning to, 'birth her inner child". To my surprise, her Midwife remained neutral and sat quietly watching and napping. At some point the mom asserted to me that I could never relate to her experience or what she was feeling so I needed to stop projecting my will onto her.

By daybreak the mother had convinced herself that she could not birth this baby without an epidural. To my great disappointment we escorted her to the hospital where she eventually birthed via cesarean.

This birth served as a lesson of patience and humility for me. The mother struggled with self-control and so did I. She had a her-story of feeling neglected, abused and molested which made it difficult for her to release the need to control her birth process. My eager passive-aggressive attempts to

5

encourage her, further disrupted her process. This birth was designed for her to learn and grow. My role was to be present and be a witness to that growth.

I realized after attending this birth that I must master self-control. My responsibility, like her Midwife, was to assume a meditative position and silently support her process by watching it unfold.

Women who are victims of sexual abuse in any capacity tend to struggle in natural, vaginal childbirth. Birth demands a woman to surrender her will to the primal forces of her body. This process can make her feel vulnerable and scared. The sensations of continuous surges and unwelcomed vaginal pressure can cause her to feel a loss of control. I witnessed a woman perform well during her labor, and upon crowning she began to scream uncontrollably while forcing her legs closed. The more we midwives persisted that she calm-down and open her legs, the more she yelled and pulled away. Simultaneously, we each released her legs and remained quiet. We could see that she was reacting irrationally. She soon composed herself, but her labor had completely stopped. This mom needed complete privacy and absolute autonomy to regain her focus and release her baby on her terms.
Be Humble!

Birth Magic Mirror

Many of us, as women, feel called to birthwork due to our own personal, traumatic birth experience. I have seen many women attracted to birthwork, unaware that they themselves have a self-fulfilling need to validate their own birth experience. If you had a traumatic birth experience, it is easy to feel triggered or reactive when re-introduced to similar and familiar circumstances. You may have developed a prejudice against obstetricians or nurses because a specific provider treated you with disrespect.

This work can be healing! It can help you to overstand the individual dynamics that are required for a woman to release her baby. However, be reminded that your role as a Birthworker is to support, and in some cases, manage the birthing process. IT IS NOT YOUR BIRTH! You cannot save a woman from her birth experience! (Non-emergent of course.) Every birth is a personal journey and individual rite of passage. It is a climax of a culmination of events, emotions, and inner-G (energy) required to bring this new being earthside.

I have witnessed some magical moments assisting families during this incredibly transformative time. I recall attending a birth as the primary alongside an senior Midwife.

August 5h, 2017: Birth is Patience

We arrived at the laboring mother's home to find seven other women. The scene was harmonious and tranquil. Each woman would synergistically offer unique support. Weather it was massage, aromatherapy, sage, chanting, singing, or drumming. We midwives would chime in from time to time and listen to baby or check her vitals. Hours passed, labor progressed and so did a thunderstorm outside. As she began to feel the urge to birth her baby, we nine women unconsciously formed a warped circle around her. As the energy of the storm increased, we anticipated birth at any minute. It felt like a spiritual scene from some recluse indigenous tribal ceremony. After several surges and growing anticipation, the mother went into a deep sleep. No one would dare to break the silence, so one by one we each would begin to nap. After about an hour, we suddenly heard keys at the front door and the knob jiggling. One would think that we would have been startled, but no one moved. Then the door crept open and their stood a silhouette of a tall and fit man with rain pouring behind him. He stepped in quietly, closed the door, removed his shoes, and briskly walked towards the circle. He moved passed us as though all he could see was her. Once by her side he kneeled and said, "I knew you were having my baby, I could feel it". Shortly after his arrival the mother birthed a healthy baby-boy. The magic in this story is that the mother did not want the father to be present. She had disconnected from him during the latter weeks of her pregnancy. She deliberately did not tell him that she was laboring. She even birthed at 41.1 weeks. Yet the father intuitively knew she was in labor and that his baby needed him.

Birthwork also has a unique way of aligning us, as supporters, with births and situations that resemble our own life experiences. In essence, we are witnessing the law of attraction. The birth scenario previously detailed was a mirror of a situation I was facing in my personal life. I was attempting to achieve a goal without the support of a significant other, though I had great support from my sister-circle. After attending that birth, I realized that this specific venture required us both and I needed him to bring forth greatness. Her shared birth experience served as a mirror for me to see what was necessary for growth and progress within my life.

This birthing magic mirror can be a powerful reflection of your life's circumstances. You may find yourself attracting problematic clients and dramatic birth experiences. This is a time for self-evaluation and self-reflection. If you have unresolved issues and birth trauma that lingers in your subconscious or conscious mind, then you are reliving this event repeatedly as your brain seeks resolution. Before pursuing your journey as a Birthworker, it is best to work through any unresolved birth trauma and life crises. Journaling, peer review, and revisiting your experience with positive-minded people can be very helpful. If you notice that you feel anxious or angry when you remember your story, then consider professional counseling. This is a necessary step prior to entering a family's sacred birthing space.
Know Thyself!!

The Abundance of Birth

As you develop your skills and grow your business, know that birth is abundant. It comes with a certain job security that I really appreciate. I realize that I can walk away from birthwork for years and return at any time knowing that people aren't going to stop having sex so babies are consistently being born. This is comforting when entering a field that at times can appear to be overpopulated with professionals.

It was many years and dozens of births later in my journey before I realized that I was only competing with myself. I invested countless hours viewing other Labor Assistants websites and appreciating their niche and talents without fully developing my own. This is partly because during that time, Doula service was a relatively new field of practice and there were not many Black women in Metro-Atlanta doing this work—I had no one to model myself after. It was challenging to affirm myself as a Doula to a community that had no idea what I was talking about. My wasband at that time was very critical of my decision to become a Doula and believed I was making a poor choice. He wasn't entirely wrong based on the odds in front of me. However, I have always been an ambitious visionary and a trail blazer. I knew that becoming a Doula was a necessary step towards me developing my inner Midwife. I eventually learned to trust my individuality and follow my interest and passions regarding birthwork. These were the intuitive processes that were guiding my journey as a Birthworker.

One of my beloved Master Teachers and mentors, Midwife Sarahn Henderson, has consistently reminded me that the Georgia Archives has record of there once being over 5,000 Midwives serving the state. These women were predominately Black and usually serving a limited geographic within walking distance from their homes. We affectionately refer to these ladies as Grand Midwives. They were indigenous to their craft and humble in their service. They practiced traditions passed down from generations of wise women. They honored the womb and respected the innate, normal, and natural ability of a woman's body to birth her baby

Today huemans are populating at an even greater number than just a hundred years ago. This is incredible considering the gross amounts of pollutants and diseases; the shortage of food and lack of planetary resources that we are constantly reminded of. We also must take account for the consistent efforts by governing bodies to control population growth. Again, we see the law of attraction at work! The more energy expressed by the self-delusional ranking powers to slow population growth,

Ironically, sociologist and anthropologist recently predicted that the White European race will become the global minority within the next 50 years due to lack of reproduction. They have an irreversible child to parent ratio that is so historically low that it has rendered their race bordering extinction within the next couple of centuries.

the more hueman beings persistently grow in astronomical numbers.

So, if you must delay your start into birthwork to tend to your family, or if you must take a sabbatical due to personal life challenges, then remember this: as long as babies are being born there is birthwork for you. Just as there are countless stars/suns within the Cosmos, each unique in size, shape, and subtle properties; be reminded that no-one can service like you, and there is a baby looking for your light....so shine!
Be Great!!

The Birth of a Business

The business aspect of birthwork by far can be the most challenging. I have seen and met with some very intelligent and brilliant healthcare providers, but their web presence and business sense were less than desirable. Fortunately for them, they have the advantage of insurance reimbursement that guarantees payment for services rendered. This reliable flow of income allows them to pay for marketing experts that can polish up their office branding and web presence while the provider focuses on their specific skill set. However, this same lack of business knowledge for an independent, Allied Birthworker can be devastating to their career.

Birthwork in any capacity is primarily an entrepreneurial field, as many Birthworker professionals own and manage their private businesses. Within the medical construct of birthwork, providers, such as Nurse Midwives and Obstetricians, are generally private contractors that apply for privileges to work within a hospital or birthing center -- in which case they are bound by the regulations and protocol of that institution. Nonetheless, these individuals are entrepreneurs that, in many settings, manage a private practice. In the case of the Obstetrician, they usually hire Nurse Midwives to work for their practice.

I have seen countless Birthworkers begin their journey of serving their communities with great zeal and optimism. These same people in some cases were very gifted and a natural at serving families within their specific scope. Sadly, their lack of business knowledge was their greatest nemesis, and they eventually abandoned their passion and returned to working a job - a place of consistent income. This has become an unfortunate trend specifically among Black Birthworkers. I believe there is this subconscious expectation that once we earn our certificate there will be a "job" type situation that we can apply for.

It is necessary to have a full game plan beyond the desire to service families. Truly evaluate your business objectives beyond credentialing. Most of these titles, such as Doula, do not require certification. It can be helpful depending on your business objectives as there are several entities and organizations offering certifications. You must know the type of Birthworker you desire to be. This will help you determine which certification or training route is correct for you before you pay hundreds of dollars.

Allied Birthworkers are charged with the responsibility and ingenuity to brand, market, and manage their business. Some will bind together and create an agency, collaboration, or partnership, whereby the funds are pooled together and used to hire accountants, billers, and marketing experts. Unfortunately, these collectives are few and far between. The bulk of us struggle to maintain our private businesses and rely greatly on networking and referrals.

Sadly, our public-school system is primarily intended to train students for the "job market". From primary school through college, we are groomed to know how to work for someone else. High schools will even teach students how to draft a resume and cover letter to apply for jobs. Granted, these skills can prove helpful, yet the skills of owning and operating a business can prove critical. Unfortunately, those of us who choose to become entrepreneurs are left to cultivate these skills independently.

The take-away here is to recognize that in choosing to become a Birthworker, you are also choosing to become an entrepreneur in some capacity. Before you enroll in a program, class, or school for developing your skills as a Birthworker, you need to first learn the basics of managing a business. Information such as, how to legitimize your business and separate your accounts for tax purposes. Know how to identify your target market and how to brand for that audience. Also know how much start-up capital you will need to invest over the first few years. These basics can help you gain the most from your Birthworker programing and have a thriving business.

I also recommend testing the waters before diving in. By this, I mean you should first explore your interest directly before investing in a training. Most allied Birthwork does not require a certification as previously explained. Therefore, it would be in your best interest to shadow a professional such as a Doula, Lactation Consultant or Childbirth Educator to learn as much as possible about the logistics of managing the business and doing the work. This experience can also help you gauge if this work is right for you before investing hundreds or thousands of dollars into a program.
Invest Wisely!

Self-Value

Self-value is a term that many Black Americans are only recently becoming acquainted with. In evaluating this phrase, we seek to overstand how it applies to us individually.

Meriam Webster Definition: Value

1 : the monetary worth of something : Market Price

2 : a fair return or equivalent in goods, services, or money for something exchanged

3 : relative worth, utility, or importance

4 : something (such as a principle or quality) intrinsically valuable or desirable

The third definition for value applies greatly to overstanding the phrase self-value. Black Americans are a people that have been greatly devalued -- displaced, discarded, defeminized, emasculated, dehuemanized, disrespected, dismissed, and discredited – for half of a millennia. Therefore, we struggle with truly identifying with self-value. Instead, we tend to place greater value on material things: clothes, cars, houses, jewelry, etc. These material gains provide a false sense of validation. I also see us use education as a means of self-validation. We strive for titles, certificates, and degrees in belief that these alphabets behind or preceding our names will grant us more value.

True self-value is rooted in self-love. The journey to self-love begins with knowing that you are worthy simply because you exist. Your existence matters! The entire Cosmos shifted to make space for your existence within this reality. Your greatness is immeasurable! Your life matters! Your health matters, and your happiness matters!

Birthwork is a service-based career. Not to be confused with servitude (slavery, bondage, subjugation). The service we market is composed of our time, energy, and expertise. The service we provide has a value. Once you know your self-value and understand the fullness of what is required of you within your scope of practice, establish a suitable fee in exchange for your service. Many of us love this work more than we love ourselves and will sacrifice ourselves to a career of servitude instead of service. It can be good business to barter fair exchange for your services. However, you always want to be certain that the exchange is complimentary to your business your livelihood.
Love Yourself!

Self-Care

Birthwork requires great amounts of time, energy, and attention. To sustain as a Birthworker, you must make intentional time for self-care. As a health-care professional you are required to provide care to your clients. If you are lacking in care, then you cannot give what you do not have. Make time for baths, massage, yoga, meditation, and peer review. Create a post-partum, self-healing regimen after each birth. It is as simple as taking a few deep breaths and having a good stretching session.

I was fortunate to participate in two Midwifery mission trips within developing countries where some days births were literally minutes apart. Even in this tense birthing climate I would intentionally step away after each birth to wash my hands and face, breath and stretch. Learn yourself well enough to know when you need a sabbatical to regroup and self-evaluate. This can help you avoid "burn out" and ensure you sustain a long and fulfilling journey serving families as a Birthworker.

Remember Yourself!

What is a Doula?

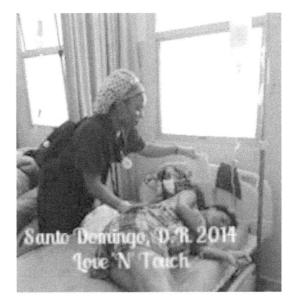

Santo Domingo, D.R. 2014
Love 'N' Touch

A service that transcends language.

Doula is a very generic term derived from Greek origins and translates as 'female slave' or 'servant woman'. I have often wondered why women would conjure up this word to describe the intimate and wholistic services provided by women for women during the maternal process. Specifically, because we overstand those words have energetic qualities and subtle implications. A Black Woman of this millennia associating herself with the word ***doula*** can be demeaning and insulting. Unfortunately, this word has spread aggressively throughout this country and extending globally — it is now identifiable and marketable. Whereas when I first became acquainted with this title in 2005, it was still very new within the southern Black community. I believe that I blindly accepted it due to my zealous spirit to answer my calling to birthwork. It would be five years later before I truly digested the full meaning of the etymology of the word *doula*. The idea began to weigh on my consciousness that I was promoting myself as a female slave and I knew my ancestors were not pleased. I immediately began to disassociate, myself with the title Doula and promote myself as a Birth Assistant. This claim brought pushback from the Midwifery community who had already coined this title for one who assisted them alongside homebirths. So, I used Labor Assistant for some time and included Doula in parenthesis or within the context for those who were familiar with the service.

From the beginning, I realized that my clients weren't concerned with my title as much as the service I provided. As a matter of fact, many of my people struggled to pronounce the word Doula and would refer to me as a Birth Coach to their friends. Now that entertainers and celebrities are popularizing the word Doula, it is becoming increasingly difficult to promote this service under a new title. The public is more aware of Doulas and are intentionally searching for them.

In reality, I am just as much responsible for promoting this demeaning word within my community as those who conceptualized it. Equally, I feel a responsibility to persist with informing my community about the etymology of the word *doula* and encourage this type of Birthworker to attach a more appropriate title to their profession.

There are many other words from dozens of other languages that can be used as a more appropriate title to describe Birth Companions or Labor Assistants. I believe it is more practical to refer to this profession as exactly what it is:

Pregnancy Care Specialist	Pregnancy Consultant
Labor Support Specialist	Labor Assistant
Postpartum Support Specialist	Postpartum Care Provider
Maternal Health Consultant	Mother Helper

The current interpretation of Doula as established by DONA, Doulas of North America:

> Doula
>> *A trained professional who provides continuous physical, emotional and informational support to a mother before, during and shortly after childbirth to help her achieve the healthiest, most satisfying experience possible.*

This definition is concise and non-threatening to the current medical profession. It clearly outlines a Doula's role as support throughout childbearing. The word Doula also sounds cute and harmless. However, I believe the scope of a Doula has evolved greatly since the inception of DONA to include a broader spectrum of services. I also recognize that the Black Community is in a current state of crisis as it relates to maternal healthcare. Our community cannot afford cute and harmless when our well-being and existence is under constant attack.

In the spring of 2018 I, in collaboration with other Birthworkers and Social Activist, trained current and aspiring Allied Birthworkers to become Maternal Health Consultants (MHC). The MHC taught the fundamentals of clinical care such as the normal ranges of blood pressures, body temperatures, urinalysis, and glucose monitoring. Knowing the normal ranges of these body systems helps to identify abnormal. Elevated glucose levels and elevated blood pressure are two primary disparities causing increased cesarean sections, and maternal and infant loss within our communities. Knowledge of these basic life-saving skills can prove to be critical in helping to ensure our maternal wellness.

Maternal Health Consultant

A care provider who optimizes maternal health outcomes with training in the fundamentals of pregnancy, labor, birth and postpartum care, using both clinical and holistic support practices. Love 'N' Touch, LLC

This definition firstly recognizes the Maternal Health Consultant as a care provider or one who provides care (personal interest, concern, responsibility). This caring person works to optimize (improve, better, correct) maternal health outcomes by utilizing both clinical and holistic (whole, complete, comprehensive) support (help, aid, assist).

Labor Assistants have always been around. They were often mothers, sisters, aunts, and other elders who provided the laboring mother with words of advice, a listening ear, a hand squeeze, or a cold compress. Today, Labor Assistants do much more than that. They are well educated support personnel who aid both parents in ensuring that the birth of their child will be an experience that meets or exceeds their expectations.

The Labor Assistant makes time to understand the needs of her client to ensure that the mother has the best possible birth experience. She is available for emotional support and helpful insight concerning the pregnancy as well as suggestions on easing minor discomforts. Prior to labor, the Labor Assistant helps the parents with preparing a birth plan that outlines the most significant concerns and choices surrounding their labor, birth, and baby. She learns comfort measures and relaxation techniques that can help bring relief to the mother during labor.

One of the most important skills of a Labor Assistant is the capability to stop the cycle of fear-tension-pain. Fear (False Evidence Appearing Real) is the anticipation of something that has not happened. Fear is rooted in ignorance because it stems from the unknown. Standard hospital procedure and protocol can leave a laboring mom with feelings of uncertainty and doubt which add to her cycle of fear. The conventional hospital labor and delivery ward has a litigious-driven etiquette of approaching a woman's labor as though it were a life-threatening illness that must be managed and controlled for the safety of herself and the unborn baby. This is a fear-based model of care, which further enhances the mother's anxiety. It is shameful that conventional hospitals employ this model with smiling faces and subtle or direct demands/threats. A Labor Assistant attempts to uproot the fears of her client by providing necessary and timely information alongside relaxation methods. She is confident in the natural process of labor and makes certain that the family is informed about their birthing options.

A Labor Assistant stays with the laboring mom throughout her labor and offers a variety of methods and means of support. Unlike other care providers such as the Obstetrician, Nurse Midwife, or Registered Nurses, who may be overwhelmed with duties that prevent their presence for the duration of a woman's labor, a Labor Assistant is there specifically for the family. She facilitates the non-clinical needs to primarily the mother, and ensures her needs are being tended to accordingly.

For these reasons it has been proven that women who received continuous support from Doulas or Labor Assistants are:

- ➢ More likely to have spontaneous vaginal births.
- ➢ Less likely to have any pain medication and epidurals.
- ➢ Less likely to have negative feelings about childbirth.
- ➢ Less likely to have a vacuum or forceps-assisted births, and Cesareans.
- ➢ More likely to have shorter labors.
- ➢ More likely to breastfeed.
- ➢ Less risks of postpartum depression in mothers.

Types of Labor Assistants

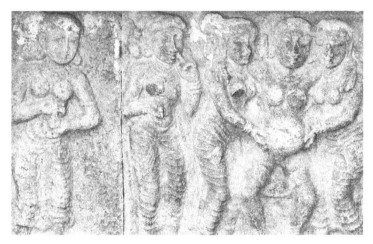

**Mural sculpture of standing-up birthing scene
on the outside wall of the Airavatesvara
Temple, 12th century CE**

September 4th, 2010: My first home birth as a Labor Assistant

There is no birth in any hospital that compares with the tranquility of a home birth where a woman is at the base of her throne. She is in a space that she knows and trusts, and most importantly she is comfortable. She is free and uninhibited to allow her body to express itself however necessary to work her baby down and out of her body.

Today I had the honor to witness and be a part of my dear friend's home birth. At her bedside I watched and served her. I tended to her needs and cared for her pains. I appreciate being a Labor Assistant......her Labor Assistant!

I was attentive and compassionate; alert and responsive; thoughtful and considerate; helpful and supportive. I helped the mom to feel secure and confident in her abilities and her power to birth her baby naturally.

I helped bring unity to the tribe, and harmony surrounding the rhythm of her birthing process. I love being a Labor Assistant!

I observed analytically as the Midwife tended to the labor and birth. She watched and guarded the gateway, ensuring a safe and delicate transition of baby. Her voice and vibe were stern and demanding, yet polite and apologetic. She was skillful and wise in her craft. I could see that her mind was filled with protocol, and it warred with her instincts to allow the miracle of birth to unfold. I love being a Labor Assistant!

Labor support allows me to be completely connected and totally detached simultaneously. I am present to help ease the discomforts and anxieties that accompany labor and birth. My attention is primarily the mom. I love being a Labor Assistant!

Initially I had only ever known of two types of Labor Assistants: Active Labor and Postpartum. These ladies usually offered special services alongside their practice, i.e., massage, aromatherapy, and yoni steaming. Some Labor Assistants will even offer non-therapeutic services, such as henna tattooing, belly casting, photography, or a birth-story. However, now I am aware of the various types of Labor Assistants, such as Fertility (Preconception), Antepartum, Bereavement, Sibling, Adoption and even a Geriatric Labor Assistant. All demographics maintain and offer the one true service, which is attentiveness. Labor Assistants are teachers, and the art of teaching begins with listening and learning your client's needs so that you can respond accordingly. A few of these demographics are explained here in more detail.

Preconception or Fertility Labor Assistant

This type of labor assistant provides informational support and guidance for families seeking to conceive naturally. They are well-trained in female reproduction, or ovulation cycles to help a woman understand tracking and charting her own fertility to identify the best window for conception. Fertility Labor Assistants also provide holistic resources and alternative therapies such as yon steaming and womb massage.

Requirements for Fertility/Preconception Labor Assistant

This labor of love does not require any certification, however there are certifying entities available both live trainings and online. Most will certify as a Full-Circle Doula or Wholistic Doula These entities typically require the following for certification:

- ➢ Become an active member of the certifying body.
- ➢ Complete an application process that usually includes references, resources, and projects.
- ➢ Complete a required reading list.
- ➢ Attend the required training or workshop (either online or live) provided by the certifying body.

Pregnancy (Antepartum) Labor Assistant

This type of Labor Assistant provides practical support to women during their pregnancy; specifically, high-risk mothers on bedrest. They also align well with teen moms, single moms, and rape victims. She provides this client with appropriate community resources and informational tools to help them prepare for birth and motherhood.

A Pregnancy Labor Assistant's greatest asset is her emotional support. She encounters women who may be feeling emotionally challenged due to feelings of confinement, isolation, abandonment, embarrassment, guilt and/or unwanted pregnancy. This Labor Assistant must be self-assured and compassionate. Counseling and life coaching skills are necessary as well to help your client with self-healing and reconciliation prior to birth.

Physical support with these moms, is pampering and grooming. These Labor Assistants will do the mother's hair, give foot massages, and provide facials. They usually offer other amenity services such as henna art and belly casting. They are also knowledgeable of different remedies for pregnancy related ailments.

Similar to Postpartum Labor Assistants, these ladies tend to do light housekeeping such as laundry and dishes, as well as meal planning and sibling care. It is very likely that the Pregnancy Labor Assistant will continue the birthing journey with their client and provide postpartum support as well.

Requirements for an aspiring Pregnancy Labor Assistant

This labor of love does not require any certification, however there are certifying entities available both live trainings and online. Most will certify as a Full-Circle Doula or Wholistic Doula These entities typically require the following for certification:

> ➢ Become an active member of the certifying body.
> ➢ Complete an application process that usually includes references, resources, and projects.
> ➢ Complete a required reading list.
> ➢ Attend the required training or workshop (either online or live) provided by the certifying body.
> ➢ Attend a Childbirth Education Class series.
> ➢ Attend a Breastfeeding Class

Labor Assistant (Doula)

"A Labor Assistant must tactfully use her Mother Wit to empower the parents and strive to maintain harmony within the laboring environment; by tuning into her instincts which enable her to conduct the natural rhythm of labor and the flow of positive energy." Birth Philosophy by Sekesa Berry

With the right support there are numerous ways a woman can labor and birth a healthy baby. I know the benefits first-hand of continuous labor support. I have given birth to four children and was fortunate to have the support of my wasbands for all of them. For each of my homebirths there was a Midwife and a Birth Assistant who provided me with continuous attention and care. This extra attention helped to empower my self-confidence and encouraged a more productive labor and birth experience. I carry this ideal with me to every birth experience I am honored to support.

A laboring mother needs to know that her pain is not in vain. She needs to feel empowered in her instincts and in her decisions. She is entitled to have as much support as she desires to accomplish the great task of bringing forth a new life. Proficient and compassionate labor support is essential for any laboring woman. This may come in the form of the support person standing by and speaking encouraging words, administering a soothing compress, giving a gentle massage, or assisting with beneficial positions. All the before mentioned techniques have been proven to ease the pains of labor and instill confidence in the mother.

When I teach relaxation classes to expectant parents, I stress the importance of relaxing in labor and the need for a woman to trust in her body's natural ability to let her baby out, instead of getting her baby out. This idea exhibits the paradox of a woman's instinct to control her labor versus her body's need for her to let go. Labor essentially is the battle between a woman's sympathetic nervous system and her parasympathetic nervous system. The sympathetic nervous system releases hormones in a woman's body that tells the uterus to contract and the parasympathetic nervous system releases hormones that tell the uterus to relax. A woman's mood has a direct influence over the intensity of this battle. The more anxiety or fear a woman has during her labor, the more tension will build in her body resulting in more pain or discomfort. Thus, great effort must be given to help alleviate the fear-tension-pain cycle that can quickly lead to the Cascade of Medical Intervention. (See diagram on page 29)

In contrast, the more relaxed and calm the mother is, the less pain she will feel. In an effort to combat this cycle, we first begin with information. The mother should be informed of the progress of her labor regularly and encouraged to manage decisions as to the direction she wants her labor to progress. She is to be comforted in whatever manner best suits her throughout her labor. She should be granted mobility and assisted with different laboring positions. The more informed and supported the mother is, the more relaxed she will feel, which brings more relief. I call this the Informed-Relief-Relax cycle or information cycle.

People instinctively will fear what they do not overstand. Education and information is the key to eliminating the fear cycle. No matter what maternal phase a woman is in, she will be met with some anxieties about the experience. By giving her knowledge, you empower her to make informed decisions rather than influenced decisions. By teaching her about what's to be expected within a certain procedure or why her body is reacting in a certain way or where to go for assistance with an issue, you help to relieve her grievances and build her confidence. This a one of the most beneficial assets of a Labor Assistant.

Requirements for an aspiring Labor Assistant

This labor of love does not require any certification, however there are many certifying entities available both live trainings and online. These entities typically require the following for certification:

> Become an active member of the certifying body.
> Complete an application process that usually includes references, resources, and projects.
> Complete a required reading list.
> Attend the required training or workshop (either online or live) provided by the certifying body.
> Attend a set number of births (average three).
> Attend a Childbirth Education Class series.
> Attend a Breastfeeding Class.

The Cascade of OB Interventions

Continuous Electronic
Fetal Heart Rate
Monitoring

Inactivity –
Confined to Bed

Increased Anxiety

False Positive
Monitor Readings

Slowed Labor

Artificial Rupture
of Membranes

Pitocin

Increased Pain

Pain Medication
and/or Anesthesia

Abnormal Fetal Heart
Rate Patterns

Use of Vacuum Extractor
and/or Forceps

Cesarean Birth

Based on The Cascade Effect in the Clinical Care of Patients by James W. Mold, MD and Howard F. Stein, PhD, *The New England Journal of Medicine*, Volume 314, Number 8 (Feb. 20, 1986), pages 512-514.

Postpartum Labor Assistant

In my experience of being a Birthworker serving the Metro-Atlanta area, few Labor Assistants have prided themselves on providing postpartum services. This is unfortunate because so many families are transplants to this area and could greatly benefit from having a postpartum Labor Assistant. Currently Georgia has one of the highest records of Maternal Mortality, with Black women leading those numbers in relation to White women 4:1. The greatest timeframe of loss is recorded as within 42-days postpartum. These women typically transition from hemorrhage, stroke, and heart failure.

> For every 13 white women who die during pregnancy or within one year of giving birth, there are 44 black women. Most of these deaths are preventable.

> "The experience of being black in America is so fundamentally different from the experience of being white in America that it translates to health outcomes," said Dr. William Callaghan, chief of the CDC's Maternal and Infant Health Branch.

> A Center for Disease Control (CDC) Foundation Report found the rate of women dying from childbirth is rising in the United States while it's dropping in other countries around the globe.

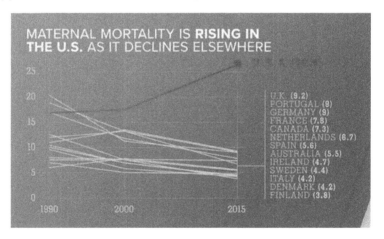

Author: Erin Peterson, Jeremy Campbell, Ciara Bri'd Frisbie, Blis Savidge, Matt Livingston
Published: 3:49 PM EDT October 13, 2018   Updated: 8:52 PM EDT October 18, 2018

Beyond yoni steaming and placenta encapsulation, though great services, moms need the basics, such as someone to watch the baby while she bathes herself, provide her with a nutritious meal, tidy up the kitchen, or simply watch her other youth while she rests for a few hours. These are the basic needs many Black American Women lack while recovering from birth, which can cause her postpartum to be more challenging. Having someone to tend to everyday seemingly mundane tasks can literally be a lifesaver.

I recall feeling the postpartum struggle after birthing my third baby. I had the luxury of living with my parents for a short time after the births of my first two babies; in fact, the second was actually birthed in their house. However, when I birthed my third baby, I lived in a different city about 80 miles away from my parents. I didn't work, and I didn't have any friends. My parents came to visit for one day and took the other two children home with them for only one week. After which they returned with my children and a casserole. That was it — I was on my own! My wasband was there but he worked 40+ hours a week. Most of the day it was me alone with a five-year-old, a three-year-old and a newborn. I would have truly appreciated having a Postpartum Labor Assistant, even if it was just for the company and someone to talk too.

The postpartum services provided by a Labor Assistant is a critical follow-up to a woman's labor and birth. Postpartum visits present opportunities for the Labor Assistant to assess for wellness and/or complications in both mom and baby. She can assist with breastfeeding, monitor how well the mom is eating and resting, and assess the mom for mental stability. These visits can range from one week to ten weeks postpartum and can be daily or weekly.

During postpartum visits, pay close attention to the family unit, particularly the mom. Watch her body language, specifically her interactions with the baby and partner. I generally schedule a minimal two-hour visit around the time of a feeding for baby. This gives me adequate time to critique the latching and positioning of the baby as well as to observe mom for any breastfeeding discomfort. Also, within this time I watch to see if the mom will eat or drink anything. I watch dad's interactions with mom and baby to better judge if he is comfortable holding baby and with assisting the mother. Dad's that are with women who are generally very organized and controlling tend to need more direction. They are accustomed to her managing the home-life, so he requires more reassurance that he can manage just as well. Some will shy away from these tasks or busy themselves to cover their uncertainties.

Ideally, a minimum of four postpartum visits should be arranged for first-time mothers. Two visits the first week after birth and two visits the second week. Veteran parents may be secure with only two visits. These visits should be about four hours or longer. The Labor Assistant should plan to either cook a meal or bring some food for the family. During the first visits the mom will most likely have several questions for you, and she may be eager to share her birth story. Remember to let her talk! It is important to allow her time for processing and recollecting her experience, particularly if you were the Labor Assistant for her birth. Ask questions about her healing such as bleeding, headaches, her bowels, and any pain or discomfort. Offer to watch the baby while she rests and assist with breastfeeding. Encourage the mother to take advantage of your visits by planning to shower, nap or have a short walk. After two weeks plan for minimal two-hour visits. These visits are more for emotional support and encouraging her to journey into motherhood. Allow time for mom to open and reveal her feelings about adapting to motherhood and parenting a new baby. Offer her community resources that encourages her to link with breastfeeding support groups, mom & baby play dates, and/or exercise programs.

The goal as a Postpartum Labor Assistant is to encourage the mother to be physically well and emotionally stable, as well as to promote competent parenting and help her to be independent of your services so that you can eventually leave her thriving well into motherhood.

Requirements for an aspiring Postpartum Labor Assistant

This labor of love does not require any certification, however there are certifying entities available both live trainings and online. These entities typically require the following for certification:

- ➤ Become an active member of the certifying body.
- ➤ Complete an application process that usually includes references, resources, and projects.
- ➤ Complete a required reading list.
- ➤ Attend the required training or workshop (either online or live) provided by the certifying body.
- ➤ Attend a Breastfeeding Class.

What is a Birth Assistant?

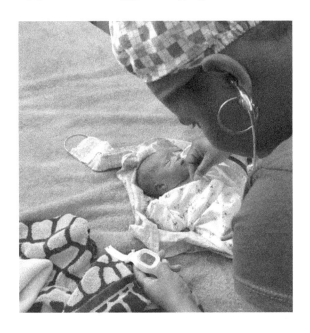

There is a saying in traditional Midwifery that is honored like a pledge by many which is, "never attend a birth alone". For this reason, a Birth Assistant has always been present in birth under different titles. There were times in our-story when that person was the birthing mother's mother, sister, aunt, husband, friend, cousin, neighbor, etc. The Birth Assistant was an extra set of hands to help support the needs of the attending Midwife. The role of the Birth Assistant has since evolved to become an extra set of *skilled* hands. In a hospital setting this would be a Labor & Delivery Nurse. In a home birth space, it can be another Midwife, a seasoned apprentice, or a woman (person) trained with fundamental clinical skills.

I served as an apprentice for about four years before being paid as a Birth Assistant. I had to learn the skills outlined here as well as demonstrate both familiarity and competency of the birthing environment. My predecessors prided themselves on being protectress of the birthing space. They were selective about who they allowed to journey alongside them. You had to prove your worth by showing commitment, perseverance, and promise. They were even more particular about paying someone to assist before they felt assured that she was competent and knowledgeable.

Once I was accepted into the ranks of Birth Assistant, I was allowed to "take-the-lead" at a birth and go ahead of the primary Midwife. I would initiate an assessment of the laboring mother and report my findings to the primary Midwife. This new role granted me an opportunity to gain more responsibility in caring for the client. I could check her vitals, time her surges (contractions), listen to her baby (check fetal heart tones), and later, as I learned to evaluate cervical change, I could also report this progress to the primary Midwife. In some cases, I would act in the capacity of a Labor Assistant to help encourage the mother's labor.

This scope of practice requires the Birth Assistant to respect the diagnosis, treatment, suggestions, and recommendations of the primary Midwife. It is important to remember that ultimately, the primary Midwife is responsible for the actions of the Birth Assistant and the outcome of this birth experience. If she sends her Birth Assistant ahead of herself to observe and care for her client, then it is from a sincere place of trust that the Birth Assistant will honor her wishes. I have witnessed Birth Assistants released from this service because their actions either disturbed or destroyed this trust relationship with the primary Midwife.

Birth Assistants are typically trained by a home-birth Midwife. In rare cases L&D Nurses will solicit their services privately to a home-birth Midwife as an assistant. A Birth Assistant is also primarily hired by Midwives for home births, and in some areas they are retained by Birth Centers.

Requirements for an aspiring Birth Assistant

This labor of love does not require any certification, however there are certifying entities available both live trainings and online. These entities typically require the following:

- Become an active member of the certifying body.
- Complete an application process that usually includes references, resources, and projects.
- Complete a required reading list.
- Attend the required training or workshop (either online or live) provided by the certifying body.
- Attendance to Childbirth education and Breastfeeding classes.
- CPR & First Aid Training.
- Neonatal Resuscitation Training.
- Assess vital signs.
- Record keeping and data entry.
- Attendance at several out-of-hospital births.
- Knowledge and operation of tools, supplies and equipment used in home birth settings such as, fetal Doppler, blood pressure monitor, thermometer, oxygen tank, urinalysis, etc.

What is an Obstetrician?

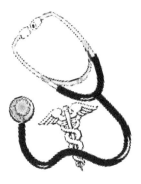

An Obstetrician is a physician specializing in obstetrics. In effort to overstand what an Obstetrician is and does in maternal health, we must first look at the root word, obstetrics.

Online etymology dictionary -Obstetric (adj.)

1742, from latin **obstetricus** "pertaining to a Midwife," from **obstetrix** (genitive obstetrics) "Midwife," literally "one who stands opposite (the woman giving birth)," from **obstare** "stand opposite to (see obstacle).

Merriam Webster Definition

Obstetrics - The branch of medical science that deals with pregnancy, childbirth, and the postpartum period.

Looking at the etymology of the word obstetrics as ***one who stands opposite the woman***, it becomes clear as to why we have dire maternal health disparities worldwide in regions where obstetricians are the authority of birthwork. Like the word *doula*, meaning female servant, slave, we must honor the tone of words. Even when we attempt to attach a different meaning to these words, the essence of it stands in truth. Words have energy, weight, and tone. This tone vibrates within the cosmos and affirms itself upon being summoned. The word obstetrics affirms to stand opposite, oppose, in opposition of the woman -- in this case the birthing woman. Whereas the word Midwife as you will see in the following chapter means ***with woman.***

Obstetricians specialize in managing pregnancy and childbirth by using a problem-solving approach known as the Medical Model of Care which focuses on the defect, or dysfunction, within the patient. These physicians have a combined discipline with gynecology, and are generally referenced as Ob/Gyn. In this book we will focus on the obstetrics discipline, however gynecology is defined below for clarity.

Gynecology – a branch of medicine that deals with the diseases and routine physical care of the reproductive system of women.

Obstetrics is a highly revered profession by Birthworkers. It represents the capstone within the hierarchy of birthwork. Obstetricians are generally a trusted community resource who helps to secure the safe growth and passage of our babies from pregnancy to birth. However, today in the United States, Obstetricians have a growing reputation of delivering impatient, impersonal, borderline neglectful service. Which explains why malpractice insurance for obstetrics averages that of a neurosurgeon, as much as $500,000 in some areas. The once male-dominated and highly sought-after career field is now on a rapid decline. So much so that hospitals nationwide are closing their Labor & Delivery departments for lack of funding and fear of litigation. Obstetrics has become a liability for hospitals that are in the business of being hospitable and making money; not losing money.

Huffington Post, June 2018

"It is an issue facing rural communities nationwide: From 2004 to 2014, 9 percent of all rural counties lost access to hospital obstetric services, and more than half of all rural counties in this country are now without a single local hospital where women can get prenatal care and deliver babies.

It is logistically challenging and expensive to staff a unit that must be ready for women day and night, and it is difficult to make enough money when there simply aren't enough women coming in. Nationally, more than half of births are funded by Medicaid, which pays doctors back at a much lower rate than private health insurance plans. In rural areas, that percentage tends to be even higher. Malpractice insurance also plays a role. Family physicians, who often deliver babies in rural areas, face higher malpractice premiums if they offer obstetric services, while hospitals may face low-volume penalties."

This decline of Obstetrical providers is leaving a serious void in rural areas across this country. I see this as the great Malcolm X said, "The chickens are coming home to roost". Obstetrics has an ugly history of career domination and standing in opposition of all other Birthworkers. Whereas it bullied, slandered and demeaned other Birthworkers politically, socially and legally, claiming to be superior to all other Birthworkers as a cleaner, safer and more dignified practice.

Witches, Nurses, & Midwives

"Witch hunts did not eliminate the lower-class women healer, but they branded her forever as superstitious and possibly malevolent. So thoroughly was she discredited among emerging middle classes that the seventeenth and eighteenth centuries it was possible for male practitioners to make serious inroads into the last preserve of female healing—Midwifery. Nonprofessional male practitioners—"barber-surgeons"—led the assault in England, claiming technical superiority on the basis of their use of the obstetrical forceps........"

"In the hands of the barber-surgeons, obstetrical practice among the middle class was quickly transformed from a neighborly service into a lucrative business, which real physicians entered in force in the eighteenth century. Female midwives in England organized and charged the male intruders with commercialism and dangerous misuse of the forceps. But it was too late—the women were easily put down as ignorant "old wives" clinging to the superstitions of the pass. "

"Throughout the latter part of the nineteenth century, the "regulars" [doctors] relentlessly attacked lay practitioners, sectarian doctors, and women practitioners in general. The attacks were linked: women practitioners could be attacked because of their sectarian leanings; sects could be attacked because of their openness to women. The arguments against women doctors ranged from paternalistic (how could a respectable woman travel at night to a medical emergence?) to the hardcore sexist."

41

Today in areas where Obstetricians honor their role intending to high-risk pregnancies and births and allow midwives to focus on normal pregnancies and births, there are overall better maternal and infant health outcomes. Obstetricians ultimately are trained surgeons. They function at their optimal in the operating room and/or in caring for women that demonstrate abnormal pregnancy, labor, and birthing circumstances. These high-risk cases need micromanaging and medical interventions. I had a client who called me to service for two of her births. She was diagnosed during pregnancy with POTS, postural orthostatic tachycardia syndrome and hypotension. She basically could not stand for long periods of time, or her blood pressure would drop dramatically, and she would faint. Her symptoms were extreme to the point that when she conceived the second child, her Ob/Gyn scolded her for risking her own life to birth another child that may or may not sustain full term. Her pregnancy required her to be on intermittent intravenous (IV) fluids, prescription meds and continuous bed rest. Now in her case we absolutely needed the care and management of an Obstetrician. There was no way I would have been comfortable tending to her needs as a Midwife. Her case is clearly out of my scope of practice.

On the contrary, I had a Labor Assistant client that was perfectly healthy. She was into fitness and eating to live. I advised her before her 37-week prenatal visit with her Obstetrician, to keep her panties on. Meaning do not allow the physician to check her cervix because it can introduce lower vaginal bacteria into and around the cervix where it doesn't belong and cause premature rupture of membranes. First pregnancy, eager and gullible, she allowed the vaginal exam. She ruptured that night with no contractions. Her Obstetrician advised her to go to the hospital. I advised her to stay home to help encourage labor with natural means. Again, eager, and gullible she and her husband went into the hospital. Almost immediately after being admitted they started her on Pitocin, which is a synthetic hormone to induce uterine contractions. This drug can be helpful when used in moderation. In most cases it makes surges more painful. This mom labored a few hours on Pitocin but soon requested an Epidural, which is a muscle relaxant that decreases pain in the body from the waist down. Nearly 12-hours later the Obstetrician enters the room and convinced the mother to have a cesarean section due to the timeline of her being ruptured increasing risks of uterine infection. There were no other associating symptoms other than this timeline upon which to perform a C-section. Now this is a case where Obstetrics was not needed. The mother should not have had a routine vaginal exam at 37 weeks. With an early rupture she needed more time to allow her body to enter labor naturally. If there were no other associating symptoms, such as abnormal vital signs, irregular fetal heart tones or meconium-stained amniotic fluid, the mother should have been encouraged to labor naturally, to see, observe, and witness her body release her baby. Medical interventions should have been delayed until deemed necessary based on any presenting associating symptoms.

I have great respect for Obstetrics and the physicians that service within this scope of practice. They save lives and help make the seemingly impossible possible every day. I believe it is necessary to adopt a title more accommodating for serving and supporting women rather than opposing them. This new title can also help to humble the "god-like", superiority complex that I have witnessed many of them project upon their patients. I believe that when the current day Obstetricians can learn to stay in their lane and play fairly with other Birthworkers, we will then see a great increase in infant and maternal wellness.

Requirements for an aspiring Obstetrician

The pathway for obstetrics in the United States is narrow. The process averages 12 years. Four years for bachelor's degree, four years medical school degree and four years residency. The basic requirements are as follows:

> A high school diploma, and a Bachelor's Degree, usually in science.

> Most students enroll in a Pre-Medicine Program which is an educational course that helps prepare them for the MCAT, and to be accepted into a Medical School. The MCAT, Medical College Admission Test, is a mandatory exam for most medical schools in the U.S.

> Attend a Medical School, preferably with a concentration in Obstetrics and women's health studies. Completion of Medical School grants a Doctorate degree, usually in General Medicine or Family Medicine.

> To achieve the title of Ob/Gyn, the education continues within a Residency Program. A Residency Program is similar to apprenticeship whereas the resident receives guided hands-on experience in gynecology and obstetrical procedures such as treatment and surgery.

> Upon successful completion of a Residency Program, a doctor can apply for a license to practice medicine within a specific state which normally entails an exam.

What is a Midwife?

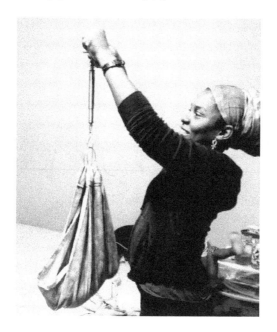

A Midwife is a woman trained to assist women in childbirth. The word derives from Old English and translates literally as "*with woman.*"

Online Etymology Dictionary - Midwife (n.)

c. 1300, "woman assisting," literally "woman who is 'with' " (the mother at birth), from Middle English mid "with" + wif "woman".

Midwives Alliance North America

Midwives are the traditional care providers for mothers and infants. Midwives are trained professionals with expertise and skills in supporting women to maintain healthy pregnancies and have optimal births and recoveries during the postpartum period. Midwives provide women with individualized care uniquely suited to their physical, mental, emotional, spiritual and cultural needs. Midwifery is a woman-centered empowering model of maternity care.....

International Definition of the Midwife
(Updated and Endorsed by the International Confederation of Midwives (ICM), June 2011)

A Midwife is a person who has successfully completed a Midwifery education program that is duly recognized in the country where it is located and that is based on the ICM Essential Competencies for Basic Midwifery Practice and the framework of the ICM Global Standards for Midwifery Education; who has acquired the requisite qualifications to be registered and/or legally licensed to practice Midwifery and use the title 'Midwife'; and who demonstrates competency in the practice of Midwifery.

The ICM definition emanates privilege and control. I completely accept that a woman who answers to the calling of Midwifery should have formal training, whether that training comes in the form of apprenticeship or institution. However, the ICM definition is exclusive to "registered" or "legally licensed". When we view our-story her-storically, we can better accept midwives as competent care providers trained with professional expertise in childbearing, birth and postpartum.

For nearly two millennia, the European colonizer has worked to demean Midwifery and dominate childbirth under the pretense of abolishing witchcraft. Much of this power struggle began with the Catholic Church during the Roman Crusades. As this patriarchal power waged war against the Muslims to secure "holy land", they simultaneously struck fear in the hearts of their European citizens, threatening persecution to anyone suspected of witchcraft. The laws created, and death penalty designed to penalize a suspect was in and of itself sick, demented, and devilish.

This is an important and pivotal point in her-story of Midwifery and women healers because during these long and brutal centuries of terror, both were suspected of witchcraft. These women were known to be freethinkers, which posed a direct threat to the agenda of the Catholic Church, whose

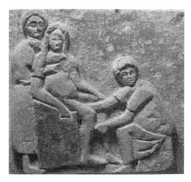

mission at that time was to subdue the people and prove dominance over all other faiths.

Witches, Midwives & Nurses

"…..the fifteenth-century witch-hunters' guidebook, *The Malleus Malificarum,* which proclaimed that "No one does more harm to the Catholic Church than midwives."

While the Europeans were in the midst of their evil, other civilizations, specifically Africans, embraced healers, midwives, and various forms of wholistic and spiritual sciences that were soon labeled as witchcraft. Those community healers were revered, welcomed, and needed. They also played a vital role in tribal decisions-making.

The Colonial State and Witchcraft: Moral Crusade or Ethnocentric Phobia.

"Pre-Colonial Times: Controlling Witchcraft the traditional way; Before colonial rule, witchcraft formed an integral part of social structure in most (if not all) traditional African societies.1 (Feireman,1990). Traditionally, the practice and threat of witchcraft was one of the numerous moral artifacts of culture for sanctioning behavior and imposing conformity. Politically, witchcraft was used to reinforce the political power of chiefs and rulers."

As the European colonizer continued to spread their racist seed and power-hungry agenda across the earth, invading Mama Africa, India, Asia, Australia, and the Americas, they also carried with them their beliefs and superstitions, as well as diseases, perversions, weapons and savagery. Within this process of oppression, enslavement and forced conformity called colonization, healers and midwives continued to be labeled as witches and deemed as threats. As a result, many of them were killed. Millions of women have been brutally murdered due to the belief of witches and witchcraft beginning as early as 500 BCE where forms of punishment and execution for witchcraft can be found within the Torah and Talmud.

Leviticus 20:27 (KJV)

27 A man also or woman who hath a familiar spirit, or who is a wizard, shall surely be put to death. They shall stone them with stones: their blood shall be upon them.

Deuteronomy 18:10 (KJV)

10 There shall not be found among you any one that maketh his son or his daughter to pass through the fire, or that useth divination, or an observer of times, or an enchanter, or a witch,

Exodus 22:18 (KJV)

18 Thou shalt not suffer a witch to live.

I have often wondered why would an all-loving, all-powerful God grant authority for one hueman to kill another? On the contray, in this book Cain killing his brother Abel was noted as the first sin and caused Cain to be cursed. However, somewhere in his-story it became acceptable to kill anyone suspected of being a witch. I digress, documentation can be found within the bible and other colonial text detailing how to test a person for sorcery or witchcraft and methods for killing them that range from drowning to stoning. For example, the float test comprised of binding the suspect with rope (rocks and stones in some cases) and tossing them into the nearest body of water to see if they would sink or float. This foolishness was based on the superstition that witches couldn't sink but rather float. The grueling result if for some reason she was able to float then she was automaticaly deemed a witch and killed. Another example was the stone test, where the accused was sandwiched between two boards and heavy stones were loaded on top. This was an insane effort to force a witch confession before crushing the person. Either method would end the life of the accused.

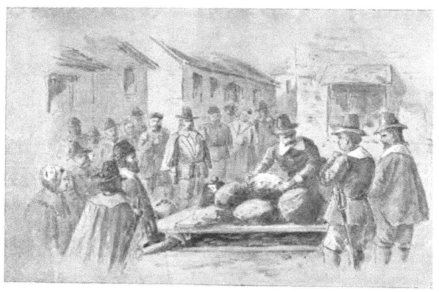

GILES COREY'S PUNISHMENT AND AWFUL DEATH.

Photo: Henrietta D. Kimball/Wikimedia

Again, it is important for us to overstand how witchcraft is linked to the near abolishment of Midwifery worldwide. As the European colonizer gained territories globally and enslaved the people of those lands, they also instilled their wicked belief systems and hatred of "free-thinking" women. There is much literature to support claims of allopathic medicine invading maternal health with direct intent to monopolize the profession within the scope of Obstetrics. What is most unfortunate is seeing the Obstetric model of care being adopted in developing countries where funding is minimal. In these areas the fading art of Midwifery is truly cataclysmic to the people. You see women traveling for miles on foot or by motorcycle to the nearest overcrowded and underfunded clinic or hospital to birth their babies. These nearby villages that once embraced the Midwife now hold in ignorance that the Midwife is unclean, uneducated and a threat to their well-being.

Logical thinking and common sense should tell the masses of people that Midwives were the first maternal health providers. Long before the words hospital, obstetrician or Midwife were adopted, women have been assisting women in childbirth for hundreds of thousands of years!! Why now, after the so called "Age of Enlightenment," have we abandoned these 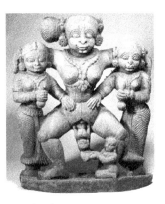 hueman customs and traditions that transcend race and ethnicity.

We people of African descent have been growing, creating, and building long before the European colonizer began to explore beyond their homeland. In order for us, as Black Americans, to survive the intentional attack on our wombs and the wombs of our sisters throughout the diaspora, we must return to customs and traditions that help aid in our continued existence. Some of these traditions include sisterhood, yoni steaming, womb massage, regular baths, herbal remedies, clean eating, homebirth, and breastfeeding. This begins with self-respect, self-care and aligning with healthcare providers that we know have a fundamental understanding of wholistic health science. Not just a specialist who is astute in one organ system or a body part (though they are needed), but a provider that comprehends the interwoven relationship of the body and mind. Because we now understand that a person's thinking can greatly impact their overall health condition. Ironically, this is common knowledge for the Traditional Midwife.

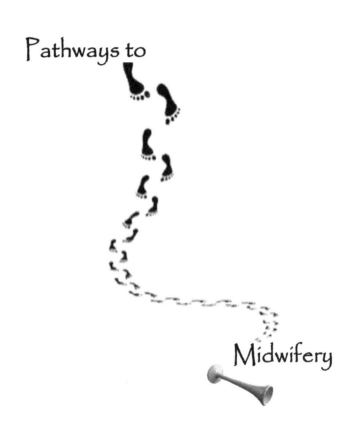

Pathways to

Midwifery

There are several pathways to becoming a Midwife. I honestly believe it is the most versatile of all other health professional schools of learning. It is also my belief that these various entry routes remain as proof that birth is a normal hueman biological process that requires minimal intervention and attention; specifically, by medical practitioners. Over the past century there has been consistent, intentional efforts made to commercialize and medicalize birth as this great emergent event that requires "trained doctors" to save the mother and/or baby. These efforts have all stemmed from a political agenda to stifle women's confidence and trust in their own bodies, then corral the masses of them into a hospital environment to satisfy a parasitic system of greed.

The many pathways to Midwifery, though unique and helpful, has also caused a hierarchy and disconnect among these healthcare professionals. It is unfortunate to see superiority complexes among those with credentials persist where there should be sisterhood. Midwifery is one of the few professions that is female dominated in a patriarchal society ruled by White middle-aged males. One would expect the fibers of Midwifery sisterhood to be strong considering the her-story of struggle. Yet the systematic war-game of "divide and conquer" is at constant play within this profession. Sometimes I fear that the credentialing, and recognition that so many Midwives lust for will result in the end of wholistic traditional and indigenous Midwifery.

As you learn the different pathways to Midwifery, it is important to keep in your mind and heart that no matter which pathway you choose, or the alphabets placed behind your name, we are all Midwives

Traditional Midwife

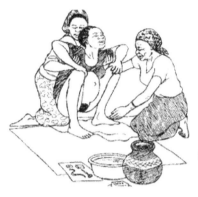

Illustration by Regina C. Faul-Doyle
Healthy Women, Healthy Mothers –
An Information Guide 2nd Ed.

" community midwife "

A Traditional Midwife is the Grand-Mother of all midwives. Her-story and legacy are as old as hueman beings. She has many titles depending on her culture, but she has always been recognized as that wise-woman. She is indigenous to her people, and in most cultures, she is highly spiritual. These women are recognized as traditional or community-based midwives. "They believe that they are ultimately accountable to the communities they serve, and in many cases to a higher spiritual power. They believe that Midwifery is a social contract between the Midwife and client, and that Midwifery should not be legislated. They also believe that women should have a right to choose a qualified care provider regardless of their legal status. Today a Traditional Midwife is described as a person who for religious, personal, and/or philosophical reasons has chosen to remain un-credentialed." (MANA)

Traditional Midwifery has a loose framework and ultimately requires the attending Midwife to have some expertise in well women's care throughout childbearing and postpartum. She relies on traditional and indigenous remedies, treatments, and methods to care for her clients. Most Traditional Midwives provide both prenatal and postpartum care for the family. In many cultures, the Traditional Midwife assumes several additional roles and services, such as the family counselor, Labor Assistant, Nanny, the Hospice, and even the Mortician. These Midwives also customarily share more time with their clients because they believe that much of their work is intuitive and requires client bonding and familiarity.

Traditional Midwives are primarily trained through apprenticeship by senior midwives. Their training and education is independent of any school and can be as rigorous or as informal as the senior Midwife requires. This pathway typically demands the apprentice to

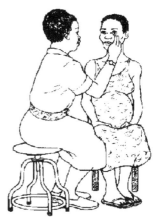

Midwife checking for anemia
Regina C. Faul-Doyle

be present for prenatals, births, and postpartum visits, while performing in the capacity of a Birth Assistant (refer to, **What is a Birth Assistant**). The senior Midwife is responsible for training her apprentice in the Midwifery Model of Care™ scope of practice as she honors it based on her beliefs, traditions, and skillset. Due to the intimate nature of the apprenticeship, the senior Midwife will usually accept an apprentice that shares similar beliefs and adheres to the morals, values, and ethics of her practice. The senior Midwife is responsible for pacing and deciding how her apprentice should learn the art of Midwifery care. Once the senior Midwife feels that her apprentice is accountable, reliable, knowledgeable, trustworthy and skill competent she will then recognize the apprentice as a peer or Midwife.

Midwives Alliance of North America

The Midwives Model of Care includes: monitoring the physical, psychological and social well-being of the mother throughout the childbearing cycle. providing the mother with individualized education, counseling, and prenatal care, continuous hands-on assistance during labor and delivery, and postpartum support.

"spiritual midwife"- Mama Oshun Nasrah

Mama Saran

The **Traditional Midwifery pathway** requires the student to seek out a preceptor for mentorship. It can be a three to five-year process or longer. The demand and cost are based primarily on the requirements of the apprenticeship. Some senior midwives require their apprentices to follow a similar learning model as the Certified Professional Midwife pathway, whereas the apprentice is responsible for attending trainings, purchasing books, and acquiring specific certifications. Other senior midwives prefer to encourage their apprentice to model them and learn entirely hands-on.

The apprenticeship model within Traditional Midwifery is as individual and unique as the people and cultures that practice it. This is both the beauty and the threat to its continued existence. As the world becomes more integrated, streamline and litigious - and governing bodies need to hold someone accountable - there seems to be no place for Traditional Midwifery.

We are All Midwives!

Direct-Entry Midwives (DEM)

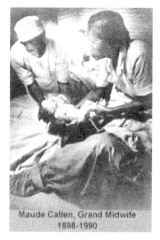

Maude Callen, Grand Midwife
1898-1990

A Direct-Entry Midwife, as defined by the Midwives Alliance of North America (MANA), is an independent practitioner educated in the discipline of Midwifery through self-study, apprenticeship, a Midwifery school, a college, or university-based program distinct from the discipline of nursing. A direct-entry Midwife is trained to provide the Midwives Model of Care to healthy women and newborns throughout the childbearing cycle primarily in out-of-hospital settings. Licensed Midwives (LM) and Certified Midwives (CM) are examples of direct-entry midwives.

state registered preceptors organization

No school
State Board of Health regulations

Midwives Alliance of North America define LM and CM as:

Licensed Midwife ~ An individual who has met specific criteria related to Midwifery by their state regulations and has been issued a license to practice Midwifery in that state.

Certified Midwife ~ The Certified Midwife (CM) credential was created to allow individuals with an undergraduate degree in a discipline other than nursing to obtain a graduate degree in Midwifery and then practice as a Midwife. They are trained and certified according to the requirements of the American College of Nurse-Midwives, take the same certification exam, and have the same scope of practice as CNMs. To date, only a few states have recognized the CM credential

The phrase direct-entry Midwifery can be confusing because it implies that a person bypassed formal education and directly entered the discipline of Midwifery and began to service families. This is exactly what the predecessors of DEM did originally! The MANA definition includes that her training can be self-study or apprenticeship, like Traditional Midwifery.

Her-story of DEM is rooted in Traditional Midwifery. In the late 1800's, DEM took form shortly after Nursing became a respectable and acceptable medical profession. Once the Nurse was ranked in the title of healthcare professional, she was then charged with the task of educating her mother, the Midwife, in the manners of the Medical Model. During the early 1900's, Nurses were hired by county health departments and were sent into rural areas throughout the United States to educate Traditional Midwives. During this time, more than half of all deliveries were conducted by Obstetricians. These deliveries were from primarily wealthy and financially secure white women. The remaining population was still very much dependent upon their local Traditional Midwife. These Midwives were predominantly Black women.

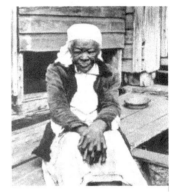

**Sibby Kelly,
Georgia Grand Midwife**

By the 1920's, county health departments began requiring for the Traditional Midwife to apply to become either registered or licensed. Many of these Traditional Midwives spoke the American English language but did not write it, so they were not permitted to apply. Others disagreed with said regulations and limitations of practice, so they either retired or concealed their practice (This equates to tens of thousands of primarily Black women). Those that did complete the trainings earned the title of Registered or Licensed Midwife. They were required to meet regularly for reporting births, ongoing trainings, and inspections. Hence the birth of Direct Entry Midwifery, DEM.

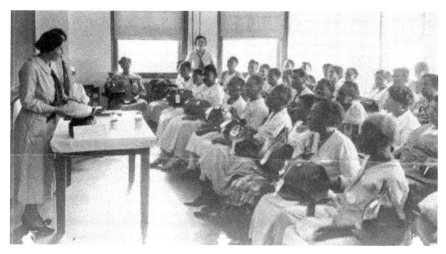

Jule Graves showing a class of midwives the contents of a model midwife bag at Florida A&M College in Tallahassee, Florida, 1935

Over time, Midwifery schools, and colleges began offering programs for DEM pathway to certification or licensure. This formal programing drew the attention of lower- and middle-class White Women. It was a form of higher learner now recognized by their society as a "respectable" career path. As these women gained interest in DEM, the face of it began to change. On until this day, White Midwives, bearing any prefix, outnumber Black Midwives an estimated 20:1.

The pathway to LM or CM depends greatly on the state you reside in. Each state regulates LM & CM independently. Some require formal education via college or accredited programming, and others allow verified apprenticeship. Some states have completely outlawed DEM and only allow Certified Nurse Midwives to practice. Other states will allow the Certified Professional Midwife to practice, while few still offer Licensure or Certification.

The LM & CM practice very similarly to the Traditional Midwife. They primarily service homebirths and offer full spectrum care. The major difference here is the credentialing and recognition that follows training. In states where Midwives are licensed, they must practice under the license of an Obstetrician. This relationship can allow them to bill insurance for service and prescribe medications. Each patient they service must first be approved by the Obstetrician for a homebirth.

Each state's health department dictates guidelines by which a LM or CM are to abide within their practice. For example, the state of South Carolina does not allow their LM's to suture, care for twin or breech births, or women over a certain age. Check the laws and regulations in your state if you are interested in pursuing this pathway to Midwifery.

We are All Midwives!

Certified Nurse Midwives

Certified Nurse Midwives are registered nurses with extended study in women's health and maternal care as it relates to preconception, pregnancy, childbirth and postpartum.

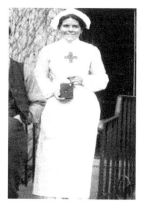

Florence Nightingale, Noted as the Founder of Nursing

Midwives Alliance of North America define CNM as:

CNMs practice in hospitals and medical clinics and may also deliver babies in birthing centers and attend at-home births. Some work with academic institutions as professors. They are able to prescribe medications, treatments, medical devices, therapeutic and diagnostic measures. CNMs are able to provide medical care to women from puberty through menopause, including care for their newborn (neonatology), antepartum, intrapartum, postpartum, and nonsurgical gynecological care

Nurse Midwifery is a part of a medical construct that regulates and authoritates the methods of Midwifery practice within an obstetrical framework. It was birthed in the United States as a part of medical reform within maternal healthcare as a tactic to combat infant mortality rates in the 1920's. (Which ironically was lower at that time with an abundance of grand-midwives in practice than it is today). Nurse Midwifery was the answer and promised to be the final solution to eradicating the Traditional Midwife problem. With Nurse Midwifery, orthodox medicine could now rank dominance over all other health-related professions.

Journal of Midwifery & Women's Health 2005
The History of Nurse-Midwifery/Midwifery Education
"Nurse-Midwifery education has existed in the United States since 1925. Originally, nurse-Midwifery was an answer to what was called the "Midwife problem" in the early 1900's. The indigenous, immigrant, and African American granny midwives, practicing at the time lacked national

handwritten annotations: "midwives", Emory Nurse Midwifery school, Frontier Nurse midwifery, (midwifery model), Northside hospital organization, a national journal for communication, access to the health care system, and legal recognition. This left them vulnerable to attacks against their profession and the work they did."

This article continues by stating, "Nurse-Midwifery emerged from the vision of public health nurses, obstetricians, and social reformers concerned about high maternal and infant mortality rates at the turn of the century. Desirous of promoting child health, they provided prenatal care for pregnant women and assisted physicians, while also supporting women during labor and birth at home. Seeking to expand their specialty by introducing nurse-Midwifery, they joined the campaign to eliminate traditional immigrant and African American midwives." **National Center for Biotechnology Information**

Nurse Midwifery has a her-story of betrayal to its grandmother, the Traditional Midwife. She rose to power without her grandmothers blessing causing a rift in the order of procession. Spear-headed by middle-class white women, they quickly disassociated from the likes of lower-class Black women and other under-privileged white women. Nurse Midwives of the roaring 1920's seized the opportunity to gain respect and recognition during a time of power-struggle and white feminism. This act of duplicity has left a whole in the fiber of sisterhood between Nurse Midwives and all other midwives.

It has only been within recent years (2016) that Nurse Midwives under American College of Nurse Midwives (ACNM) came together with the National Association of Certified Professional Midwives (NACPM), and other nationally recognized organizations to form a coalition known as the US Midwifery Education, Regulation, & Association (USMERA). This entity was formed in attempt to unify credentialed midwives and establish standards of education and practice

Nurse Midwives are advanced in the craft of Midwifery. They have a core foundation of nursing, where they learn the clinical aspects of medical practice, healthcare, and hospital procedure. This extended knowledge grants Nurse Midwives a broader scope of practice than any other field of Midwifery, awarding them skills in phlebotomy, gynecology, pharmacology, and some obstetrical practices such as forceps and vacuum extraction. However, Nurse Midwives are held to a greater standard of accountability by both hospitals and Obstetricians which can limit their ability to provide the full Midwifery Model of Care™ (see page 53). Within this model of care, midwives are expected to provide, "continuous hands-on assistance during labor and delivery, and postpartum support." Nurse Midwives working in hospital settings, with multiple patients are rarely allotted time to provide continuous assistance to one woman. This gap in care is where the Labor Assistant is greatly needed most.

Nurse Midwives in the United States rarely own private practice and generally work in collaboration and under the supervision of Obstetricians. These partnerships and collaborations have resulted in two types of Nurse Midwives that we as allied birth professionals refer to as Medwives and Midwives. If the Nurse Midwife is partnered with an Obstetrician who is medically-minded, surgically motivated and harbors fears of unpredictable, natural childbirth, then this method of practice becomes instilled in the Nurse Midwife. Whereby she will negate the core aspects of Midwifery, which are to trust birth and only intervene when necessary. Instead, the Medwife can be found micro-managing and excessively augmenting the labor process; essentially operating from a space of fear.

Nurse Midwifery is a growing career field due to the decline of Obstetricians. Many women are answering their calling to birthwork through this formal educational pathway. Nurse Midwifery is certainly the most defined pathway in terms of schooling. **There are two options for becoming a Nurse Midwife, yet both must be initiated with a nursing degree.** This nursing degree can either be License Practitioner Nurse (LPN) or Registered Nurse (RN).

> ➢ High school diploma and an Associate or Bachelor's in nursing.
> ➢ Typically work at least one year as an RN, preferably with an in OB/Gyn practice.
> ➢ Graduate from a master's or a doctorate program accredited by the Accreditation Commission for Midwifery Education (ACME)
> ➢ Must pass the American Midwifery Certification Board (AMCB) exam.

The second pathway to Nurse Midwifery is called the **Bridge program.** Here a Nurse with an Associate Degree, ADN, can earn a Master of Science in Nursing, MSN, with a nurse Midwifery focus. Essentially skipping the BSN step, as this program allows one year to 18 months of programing and MSN-level coursework.
We are All Midwives!

Certified Professional Midwives

The Certified Professional Midwife (CPM) was birthed out of the 1970's by liberal White Women identifying as Hippies. These socially defiant women were re-connecting to nature and re-claiming the autonomy of their bodies. They were embracing womanhood, sisterhood and motherhood, with a more self-directed, unconventional and free-thinking attitude. As such, many of them chose to birth their babies at home either with Traditional Midwives or with more experienced friends.

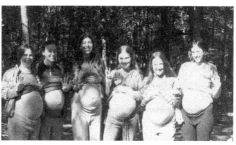

Birth Story: Ina May Gaskin & The Farm Midwives ©

"Spiritual midwifery" Book

Certified Professional Midwives in the United States: An Issue Brief From NARM, MEAC, NACPM and MANA, June 2008

A new generation of direct-entry midwives emerged in the 1970s to serve those women who were rediscovering normal birth and choosing to give birth at home. What began as a grassroots movement almost forty years ago has evolved into a body of professionals with a national identity. This professionalization began in 1982 with the founding of the Midwives Alliance of North America (MANA), an organization that brought together midwives from all backgrounds who were committed to unifying and strengthening Midwifery.

By November 1991, MANA developed the Interim Registry Board (IRB) Registry Examination to measure the core competency of an aspiring Midwife and was officially administered to Direct-Entry Midwives that same year. Over the next few years and many convenings with Nurse Midwives, it was decided that direct-entry midwives needed to develop their own credentialing and accrediting mechanisms (MANA). In 1992 IRB

Juantina - Kentucky Birth center

incorporated a non-profit titled National Alliance of Registered Midwives (NARM) and together, with MANA, they birthed the Midwifery Education Accreditation Council (MEAC). The job of MEAC was to guide the development of the direct-entry Midwife certification process. It was then decided that the certification process would require two components: education and certification (MANA).

> "The educational portion consisted of a specified clinical component as part of the educational evaluation and documentation of clinical skills with preceptor verification of proficiency. The certification verification was comprised of an extensive Written Examination that would be based on a Job Analysis survey that would determine the essential body of knowledge and skills necessary for safe and competent entry-level, out of hospital Midwifery practice." (MANA)

The first CPM was issued in November of 1994 which marked the beginning of the NARM Certification Process The educational process for NARM credentialing can be completed in three different pathways:

> "......graduation from a MEAC or AMCB (formerly the ACC) accredited program, through legal recognition from a state or province that has been evaluated for educational equivalency from NARM, or through the Portfolio Evaluation Process (PEP). (MANA) The PEP application evaluates education through apprenticeship, special circumstances, or international programs, and includes verification of supervised experience." (NARM)

Now here is where achieving credentialing for Midwifery becomes daunting and discouraging for many Women of Color living in the United States. Each of the educational pathways detailed above presents with serious considerations based on geographical location. Since the intentional removal of Traditional Midwives, some areas have few to no Black CPM's. This makes finding a qualifying preceptor for us challenging. Specifically, if we desire to service women in our communities and learn the traditions, cultures, and values of our people. Affordability is another hindrance for us. Federal grants currently do not pay for MEAC programs and scholarships are scanty. Those few of us who have managed to commit to the requirements of the PEP process struggle to commit to several years of attending prenatal visits and births as an unpaid or underpaid apprentice. We often find ourselves attempting to juggle a conventional job alongside our families and the obligations of an apprenticeship.

Meanwhile, White CPM's have more than tripled over recent decades, leaving an estimated ratio of Black to White CPM's of 1:20. According to the 2016 NARM Annual Report, there was recorded 3004 CPM's in the country. Of that number approximately 150 of these ladies are Black

To better understand this great disproportion, we must consider the timeline for Black Americans as it parallels to the timeline of developing the certification process for credentialing Direct-Entry Midwives. During the 1960's and 70's Black Americans were consumed with organizing, marching, fighting, standing, and sitting for Hueman Rights and Civil Rights. Meaning the right to be treated as hueman and the right to be recognized as an American citizen.

> **Hueman rights** are rights inherent to all hueman beings, regardless of race, sex, nationality, ethnicity, language, religion, or any other status. Hueman rights include the right to life and liberty, freedom from slavery and torture, freedom of opinion and expression, the right to work and education, and many more. Everyone is entitled to these rights, without discrimination. (United Nations)

> **Civil Rights** refers to the basic rights afforded, by laws of the government, to every person, regardless of race, nationality, color, gender, age, religion, or disability. This refers to such rights as equal citizenship, equal protection under the law, and due process. (LegalDictionary.net)

By the early 1970's Black Americans were grieved for murdered leaders and crumbling organizations. We were struggling to adapt to newly acquired integration policies, affirmative actions and voting rights. Only to be met with a new sabotage -- recreational drugs. Drugs that "wreck" our creative abilities. Our communities suddenly became flooded with all types of new recreational drugs: PCP, LSD, Quaaludes, and heroin, to name a few. The 1970's drug

> It is mind-baffling that impoverished, low-income Black and Brown subsidized-living communities can somehow afford elaborate weaponry such as the Street Sweeper™ and AK-47™.

epidemic was devastating to the Black family unit. To this day in 2018 we have yet to recover. It divided Black families, demoralized Black cultural values and left many Black family homes fatherless due to abandonment, imprisonment or death. No sooner than we attempted to unite in the 1980's, our communities were hit with crack cocaine, an abundance of guns and violent gangs. Our residential neighborhoods and schools became war zones in some areas.

The inequities were compounded by the unforgettable "War on Drugs" in the 1990's that enforced the "three strikes" bill on a people that were already challenged by an unjust legal system. This three strikes law imprisoned millions of Black and Brown men and women between 1994 (the year of the first CPM) and 2004 -- more than in the history of the United States. Unfortunately, this cycle continues today.

All awhile these dynamics were prevailing, in Black American culture we were losing our Traditional and Grand Black Midwives. They were transitioning with few that they could pass on their wisdom and knowledge to. One of the last of these women was a Traditional Midwife in Alabama, Margaret Charles Smith, known for her book Listen to Me Good: The Life Story of an Alabama Midwife, and catching over 3000 babies. Margaret transitioned in November of 2004.

The strategic and intentional marginalization of Black and Brown Americans through economics, education, healthcare, politics, and litigation has greatly derailed our collective progress in this country and hindered our growth in many ways, including the Midwifery profession.

The CPM pathway(s) has proven not to be the best fit for Black American women for many of the before mentioned reasons. I have seen many of us attempt this pathway, only to detour into Nurse Midwifery instead. As I stand on the shoulders of Grand Midwives and watch the shift of allegiance from traditional customs to medical conventions among my people, I do wonder what the future of Midwifery (with-woman) holds for us.

Requirements for an aspiring Certified Professional Midwife

As mentioned before there are three identified pathways to fulfilling the educational process to CPM. Each process ends with the required NARM Written Examination. Pathways listed below are not in any significant order.

a. **School Pathway requires graduation from a MEAC or AMCB accredited program.**
b. **Legal recognition from a state or province that has been evaluated for educational equivalency from NARM.**
c. **Portfolio Evaluation Process (PEP) application evaluates education through apprenticeship, special circumstances, or international programs, and includes verification of supervised experience.**

The PEP process is the most liberal and most difficult (in my opinion) of the above listed pathways. An information booklet detailing the requirements, didactics and documentation can be found on the NARM website.

We are All Midwives!!

Closing Remind-hers

Conventional or allopathic medicine has greatly hindered the community it serves, most notably Black Americans. The system arrogantly claims to be the Primary Care Provider (PCP) and many Black Americans surrender their health-care to this system that does not care. Remember that words have energetic qualities and subtle implications. When one other than the "self" is appointed as primary then the subconscious mind (self) will cease to care about self and neglect self-care. The subconscious mind charges the person appointed as primary (first, chief, leader, parent, guardian) healthcare provider, with managing personal health. If this appointed person is other than the self, then the person will lack care (health, wellness) -- hence the common phrase, "I don't care".

It is of vital importance to discern words and their implications. This helps us process information more accurately which allows us to perform with greater intention. Simply put, we must say what we mean; and mean what we say. The governing bodies and the financial institutions are very intentional and strategic in both words and action.

This information era, that we are each blessed to be present in, has removed the cloak away from hiding several generations of intentional attacks on Melanated people and the Black womb. It is a dreadful and ugly picture of sterilization, experimentation, eugenics, and genocide through manipulation, commercialization, and bio-chemical means. Most of which today we, as Black Americans, willingly participate through trusting a medical system that does not care about our health.

> Black women globally are being attacked. This attack is a covert one and often times waged under the banner of "feminism" and "women's liberation" but in fact it has everything with destroying Black women's health, fertility, and wombs. This attack is being waged for purposes of imperialism, population control/eugenics, and profit. Billionaire industries like Big

Pharma, the Medical Monopoly, Big Energy, Monsanto, and huge chemical companies are involved in this bio-chemical war. The US government and eugenics organizations like Planned Parenthood are also major players in this bio-chemical war to destroy Black women as well. This war has been secretly waged for several decades and as a result, millions of Black women have been sterilized, millions have had their wombs removed, millions have been killed by modern medicine, millions have been poisoned by toxic chemicals, and tens of thousands have been killed or maimed during hospital births. Black women now also have the highest rates of diabetes, obesity, fibroids, and breast cancer. The weapons and warriors in this war are the government, Bill Gates, the Rockefeller Foundation, billionaire population control eugenicists, the CDC, doctors, hospitals, feminists, OB/GYNs, modern medicine, Black hair care products, vaccines, pharmaceutical drugs, birth control, drinking water, plastic bottles, and food.   *Dr. Curtis Duncan*

This is a controversial, yet strong sentiment expressed by Dr. Curtis Duncan. It reveals the ugly truth that Black women have been continuously and intentionally subjected to poor healthcare. Now more than ever, there is a great necessity for Black Birthworkers to service our communities and become protectors of the Black womb.

I believe that babies are the return of our ancestors, grandparents, and great-grandparents. In the tradition of indigenous birthing, we must become gatekeepers and honor the birthing mother (the vessel, the vortex, the goddess) with healthy and safe options; respectful and caring providers; and gentle Love 'N' Touch.

Midwife Sekesa Berry, Author

Sekesa Berry is a loving mother of four children and a community mother to many. She has serviced her community for over a decade as a Labor Assistant (Doula) and a Lactation Consultant. Now serving as a Traditional Midwife, she is also the founder and director of the Atlanta Doula Collective non-profit organization, and curator of the Maternal Health Awareness Training a.k.a. the Advanced Doula Skills

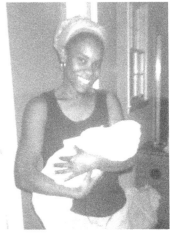

My First Catch 2008

Training. Sekesa has achieved a level of recognizable service to her community working nearly two decades with several non-profit organizations both locally and nationally in effort to empower families with evidence-based information and wholistic options for optimal maternal health outcomes..

"I have known since the age of 13 that I wanted to help mommas have babies. As an adolescent I was directed towards Obstetrics by my elders but once in college I quickly learned that it was not for me – I did not want to cut on women. The medical profession did not resonate with my spirit. It wasn't until my first homebirth experience that my passion for Midwifery was confirmed and ignited. I was free to labor and birth my baby with my body as my guide and my midwives as my support. This experience marked as a pivotal point in my life. It revealed another world of possibilities to me aside from obstetrics and nursing. I learned that with the right support there are countless ways women can labor and birth a healthy baby as well as create beautiful birth stories."

Abundant Blessings

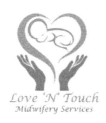

Love 'N' Touch
Midwifery Services

Bibliography

Arkutu, Ananie. Healthy Women, Healthy Mothers. Family Care International, Inc., 1995.

Bar-Ilan, Meir. "Witches in The Bible And In The Talmud." #39&פרוס; מאיר בר-אילן: Witches in The Bible And In The Talmud, faculty. biu.ac.il/~barilm/articles/publications/publications0038.html.

Burst, H. V. "The History of Nurse-Midwifery/Midwifery Education." The Journal of Midwifery & Women s Health, pp. 50: 129-137, doi:10.1016/j.jmwh.2004.12.014.

Dawley, K. "Origins of nurse-Midwifery in the United States and its expansion in the 1940s." Journal of Midwifery and Womens Health, Mar-Apr. 2003 pp. 48(2):86-95. National Center for Biotechnology Information, www.ncbi.nlm.nih.gov/pubmed/12686940.

Duncan, Curtis. "The Bio-Chemical War on the Black Womb: The Secret War on Black Women's Health and Fertility." Curtis Duncan. 30 July 2016, www.drcurtisduncan.com/2016/07/the-bio-chemical-war-on-black-womb.html. Accessed 12 July 2018.

Ehrenreich, Barbara, and Deirdre English. Witches, Midwives & Nurses. second ed., Feminist Press, 2010.

Mesaki, Simeon. "Tanzania Zamani - The colonial state and witchcraft: moral crusade or ethnocentric phobia - The case of British colonialism in Tanganyika." Historical Association of Tanzania/History Department, vol. 3, no. 1, 1997, pp. 50 – 71, hdl.handle.net/10520/AJA08566518_20.

Pearson, Catherine, and Frank Taylor. "Rural Maternity Wards Are Closing And Women's Lives Are On The Line." The Huffington Post, TheHuffingtonPost.com, 4 June 2018, www.huffingtonpost.com/entry/maternity-wards-closing-mission_us_59c3dd45e4b06f93538d09f9.

Peterson, Erin, et al. "Why Childbirth Is a Death Sentence for Many Black Moms." WXIA, 13 Oct. 2018, www.11alive.com/article/news/investigations/mothers-matter/why-childbirth-is-a-death-sentence-for-many-black-moms/85-604079621.

CPSIA information can be obtained
at www.ICGtesting.com
Printed in the USA
LVHW050306311222
736049LV00002B/455

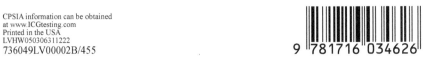